Ketogenic Recipes to add Variety to your diet

Choosing the Ketogenic Diet is most definitely a lifestyle choice. There are tremendous benefits to choosing this way of eating, which becomes a way of life. There are always obstacles that we come across whether it be limited ingredients and/or a limited budget!

There are a few different Keto guidelines as far as what should and should not be included in the eating plan. In this book, there are recipes for every budget. Keto is really quite basic and the foods can get a little "boring", here's to help create a little party in your mouth!

So, without sounding to preachy or mundane, here is what you picked up the book for.. RECIPES:

Paleo Egg Muffin Puffs

- **Eggs (6)**
- **Nitrate Free Shaved Turkey (6 slices)**
- **Sliced Spinach (½ cup)**
- **Red Pepper (3 tablespoons)**
- **Mozzarella Cheese Light**
- **Fresh Basil (optional)**
- **Red Onion (2 table spoons, finely chopped)**
- **Salt & Pepper**

Directions :

1. Preheat the oven to 350°;

2. Slice the spinach, red onion, red pepper and basil and grate the mozzarella cheese.

3. Spray a nonstick muffin tin with olive oil spray ;

4. Gently drape the piece of turkey in one of the muffin cups so that it rests on the bottom and the sides of the tin to make a larger cup.

5. Carefully crack an egg and pour it into the turkey cup.

6. Add a little bit of sliced red onion, spinach, red pepper and cheese on top of the egg.

7. Add some fresh basil and grind a bit of fresh pepper and salt onto the egg.

8. Put the muffin tin in the oven and bake until eggs are set and the whites are opaque, about 10 minutes for a runny yolk and closer to 15 minutes for a harder one. Keep in mind that the egg muffins will cook for a bit longer when you take it out of the oven.

GUACAMOLE

Ingredients

- **4 Avocados**
- **1 Small Onion**
- **2 Tomatoes**
- **1 Jalapeno**
- **1 Tbsp Lime or Lemon Juice**
- **½ tsp Salt**
- **½ tsp Cumin**
- **½ tsp Salt**
- **½ tsp Cayenne Pepper**
- **1 Tbsp Minced Garlic**

Instructions

1. **Start by peeling and chopping the Avocados**
2. **Place the Avocados in a large bowl and toss with the lime or lemon juice**
3. **Add the spices and mash the Avocados with a potato masher**
4. **Add the Jalapenos, onions and tomatoes and mix again**
5. **Store at room temperature for 1 hour before serving to allow juices to blend.**

Chorizo and Chicken Soup

Ingredients

- **4 Lbs Cut up Chicken**
- **1 Lb Chorizo**
- **4 Cups Chicken Stock**
- **1 Cup Heavy Cream**
- **1 Can Stewed Tomatoes**
- **2 Tbsp Minced Garlic**
- **2 Tbsp Worcestershire Sauce**
- **2 Tbsp Frank's Red Hot Sauce**
- **Garnish with Shaved Parmesan and Sour Cream**

Instructions

1. **Brown chorizo in a skillet**
2. **Layer the ingredients into the crockpot starting with the Chicken Thighs (raw), Chorizo then the remaining ingredients**
3. **Cook on high for 3 hours in crock pot then 30 more minutes on low or cook on stove starting on Medium High for an hour- just make sure chicken is not pink.**
4. **Garnish with Shaved Parmesan and Sour Cream!**

Bacon Wrapped Jalapeno Poppers

Ingredients

12 Fresh Jalapenos

8 oz medium cheddar cheese

8 oz cream cheese

package of bacon

Directions

1. Slice off the top of each jalapeno then slice them in half the long way.
2. Scoop out the jalapeno seeds and throw away.
3. Stuff each jalapeno side of the jalapeno with cut up cheddar cheese and cream cheese.
4. Wrap the bacon around the jalapeno with cheese.
5. Place on pan and put in 350 degree oven for a min of 30 minutes, until cheese is melted.
6. Let cool a little bit and enjoy!

Chicken Avocado Casserole

Ingredients

- 8 Boneless Chicken Thighs, cooked
- 4 Small Avocados
- 1 Medium Onion
- 1 Medium Pepper
- 8 Oz. Sour Cream
- 8 Oz. Cheddar Cheese
- 1 Tbsp Frank's Red Hot
- Salt and Pepper to taste

Instructions

1. Preheat oven to 350 F
2. Start by cooking the chicken thighs, for this recipe I had them already cooked, but just bake at 350 for 1.5 hours covered with some water or cube and pan fry until juices are clear
3. Peel avocados, cut in half, and slice into thin strips
4. Grease a baking dish and line the bottom with avocado slices, reserve any extra
5. Cut the peppers and onions into strips and pan fry until caramelized
6. Add the chicken into a large bowl and flake apart
7. Add remaining ingredients, including any extra avocado, and mix
8. Spoon mixture over the avocado slices
9. Bake for 20 minutes

St. Louis Ribs- Keto Style

Ingredients

- **2 racks of St. Louis Ribs (6.72 lbs)**
- **2 Tbsp Paprika**
- **1 tsp Stevia**
- **1 Tbsp Garlic Powder**
- **1 Tbsp Salt**
- **½ Tbsp Pepper**
- **½ Tbsp Ground Ginger**
- **½ Tbsp Onion Powder**
- **¼ Tbsp Cayenne Pepper**
- **2 Oz. Dijon Mustard**

Instructions

1. **Preheat oven to 225 degrees**
2. **Using a sharp knife, remove the membrane on the back of the ribs if it is present**
3. **Mix together all of the spices**
4. **Spread mustard all over the ribs**
5. **Rub the spice mixture into the meat**
6. **Place the ribs on a foil lined sheet**
7. **Bake uncovered for 60 minutes**
8. **Tent the meat with some aluminum foil and cook for 3.5 more hours or until the internal temperature reaches 180 degrees, turning after 2 hours**
9. **Remove the foil and broil on high for 5 minutes to develop a good crust**
10. **Cover and let rest for 10 minutes**

Coconut Shrimp

Ingredients

- **Shrimp**
- **12 Large Shrimp**
- **30 g Shredded Coconut**
- **15 g Flaked Coconut**
- **90 g Mayo (6 Tablespoons)**
- **45 g Unsweetened Coconut Milk (3 Tablespoons)**
- **1 egg yolk**
- **Dip**
- **60 g Mayo (4 Tablespoons)**
- **10 ml Chili Garlic Sauce (2 tsp)**
- **5 ml Unsweetened Lime Juice (1 tsp)**

Instructions

1. **Thaw and dry the shrimp**
2. **Mix together the rest of the shrimp ingredients**
3. **Coat the shrimp in the mixture**
4. **Drop the shrimp into the fryer and cook until golden brown**
5. **Mix the dip ingredients together**
6. **Serve!**

5-Layer Keto Dip

Ingredients

- **20 Oz Guacamole**
- **4 Oz Cream cheese**
- **4 Oz Mayonnaise**
- **8 Oz Sour Cream**
- **2 Tablespoons Taco Seasoning-- recipe follows**
- **16 Oz Salsa**
- **10 Oz Cheddar Cheese, Shredded**
- **4 Oz Green Onions, Diced**

Instructions

1. **Start by combining the cream cheese, mayo, sour cream and seasoning**
2. **Mix until smooth**
3. **Chop up the green onions**
4. **(Layer 1) Using a medium sized casserole dish, start by spreading out the guacamole on the bottom**
5. **(Layer 2) Then carefully spread the sour cream mixture over top of the guac**
6. **(Layer 3) Now spread the salsa over the sour cream mixture**
7. **(Layer 4) Add the cheese**
8. **(Layer 5) Top with green onions**
9. **This is best if you let it sit in the refrigerator for at least an hour and up to 24 for the flavors to intermingle**

Homemade Taco Seasoning

Ingredients

- 1 part chili powder
- 1 part ground cumin
- 1 part garlic powder
- 1 part onion powder
- 1/4 – 1/2 part crushed red pepper

Directions

- Mix all the spices together and store in an airtight container. I store mine in the freezer!
- Use sparingly. Or liberally!

GINGER BEEF

Ingredients

2 sirloin steaks, cut in strips

1 Tblsp MCT Oil or Butter

1 small diced onion

1 clove crushed garlic

2 diced tomatoes *optional

1 teaspoon ground ginger or grated fresh ginger

4 Tblsp Bragg's apple cider vinegar

Sea Salt and Pepper to taste

1. **Place the oil in a large skillet and brown the steaks over medium-high heat.**
   2. **When both sides are well-seared, add the onion, garlic and tomatoes *optional.**
   3. **In a bowl, stir ginger, salt and pepper into the vinegar. Add mixture to skillet, stir to combine.**
   4. **Cover the skillet, turn the heat to low, let the dish simmer until mixture evaporates.**
   5. **Serve and enjoy!**

Buffalo Crockpot Chicken

Ingredients

- **6 Frozen Chicken Breasts**
- **1 Bottle Frank's Red Hot**
- **2 T Ranch Mix-- recipe follows**
- **3T Butter**

Instructions

1. **Put the chicken in the crockpot**
2. **Pour the hot sauce over chicken and sprinkle ranch over top**
3. **Cover and cook on low for 6 hours**
4. **Shred, add butter, and cook on low for 1 hour uncovered**

Ranch Mix Recipe

1/2 cup <u>dry buttermilk</u>

- **1 tablespoon <u>dried parsley</u>, crushed**
- **1 teaspoon <u>dried dill weed</u>**
- **1 teaspoon <u>onion powder</u>**
- **1 teaspoon dried onion flakes**
- **1 teaspoon sea <u>salt</u>**
- **1/2 teaspoon <u>garlic powder</u>**
- **¼ teaspoon <u>ground pepper</u>**

Directions:

1. **Combine all ingredients in a blender.**
2. **Blend at high speed until smooth.**
3. **For salad dressing, combine 1 Tablespoon of mix with 1 Cup of mayonnaise and 1 Cup of Organic Milk.**
4. **To use dry, 1 Tablespoon equals an envelope of Ranch dressing mix.**

Spinach, Shallots and Bacon

- **16 ounces raw spinach**
- **1/2 cup chopped white onion**
- **1/2 cup chopped shallot**
- **1/2 pound raw bacon slices**
- **2 tablespoons butter**

Directions:

1. Slice the bacon strips across in small narrow pieces.
2. Start a large skillet with butter.
3. Add the chopped onion, shallots and bacon. Saute for about 15 -20 minutes or until the onions have started to carmelize and the bacon is cooked.
4. Add the spinach leaves.
5. Saute on medium heat, stirring occasionally, and making sure you turn over the leaves up from the bottom so that the top leaves also make contact with the hot skillet, as the whole pile cooks down. This also mixes in the bacon and onions.
6. Cover the skillet and let the spinach mixture steam for about 5 minutes. Stir again and repeat until the spinach is wilted and cooked.

Creamed Spinach

- 16 ounces raw spinach
- 1/2 cup chopped white onion
- 1/2 cup chopped shallot
- 1 clove garlic, minced
- 2 tablespoons butter
- 1/2 cup of heavy cream
- 1/4 teaspoon nutmeg
- Salt and pepper to taste

Directions:

1. Start a large skillet with butter.
2. Add the chopped onion, shallots and garlic. Saute for about 5-10 minutes or until the onions have softened.
3. Add the spinach leaves.
4. Saute on medium heat, stirring occasionally, and making sure you turn over the leaves up from the bottom so that the top leaves also make contact with the hot skillet, as the whole pile cooks down. This also mixes in the onions.
5. Cover the skillet and let the spinach mixture steam for about 5 minutes. Stir again and repeat until the spinach is wilted and cooked.
6. Add the cream and nutmeg and stir to mix. Cook for about 3-4 minutes more to reduce the liquid and thicken the cream.
7. Add salt and pepper to your taste.

Triple Coconut Keto Cupcake

Ingredients

- ½ Cup Vanilla-flavored protein powder
- 2/3 Cup Coconut flakes, unsweetened
- 1 Cup Coconut milk, unsweetened
- 4 Tbsp Coconut oil
- 2 Tbsp Psyllium husk
- Dark chocolate min. 85% cocoa

Directions

Step 1

In a medium sized bowl, mix well the protein powder (we used a nearly zero carb variety), the coconut flakes, and the psyllium.

Step 2

Add the coconut mil and the coconut oil (liquefy it first if needed) into the dry mix and blend very well.

Step 3

Divide the batter into cupcake forms, it should be just enough to fill 7 standard size cupcake forms. We used silicone moulds but, since you will not need to bake these cupcakes, it's ok to use paper cupcake forms.

Step 4

Crush and melt the chocolate and decorate the cupcakes to your liking.

Step 5

Place the cupcakes in the freezer for about 30 minutes. They don't need to deep freeze, we only want for them to achieve a more solid consistency.

Step 6

Remove cupcakes from the freezer and store in the refrigerator, or at least in a cold place. Coconut oil melts at just 24 degrees Celsius (75 F) so have that in mind if you're taking cupcakes to work or anywhere else you might not have a chilled place to store them.

The Ultimate Keto Bomb

Ingredients

- **2 Oz. Coconut Oil**
- **1 Oz. Cream Cheese**
- **½ Oz. Torani Sugar Free Vanilla Syrup**
- **1 teaspoon Cocoa Powder**
- **2 Oz Dark Chocolate (I Used 85%)**
- **8 Drops Stevia Drops**
- **2 Oz. Almond Butter**

Instructions

1. **Combine all the items except the almond butter and microwave for 30 seconds**
2. **Stir the ingredients, if the chocolate is not fully melted, microwave again and continue stirring**
3. **Pour a base layer into the mold you're using**
4. **Then using a spoon and place a dollop of Almond Butter in the center**
5. **Fill the rest of the mold to the top**
6. **Freeze until the chocolate hardens, when hard push them out of the mold**
7. **Store in the fridge**

Ice Cream Pops

Ingredients

Can of Coconut Milk

¼ cup ceylon cinnamon

1/2 teaspoon Stevia TWICE

Coconut Oil

Directions

1. Take ½ of the can of coconut milk, put in bowl and using a mixer, add in ½ teaspoon Stevia. Mix and set aside.
2. Take the other ½ of the can of coconut milk, add the ceylon cinnamon and the other ½ teaspoon of Stevia.
3. Take your molds and layer the 2- coconut milk mix and the coconut milk and cinnamon mix. Sporadically, add drops of coconut oil about halfway through to add a little crunch to the popsicles.
4. Freeze and enjoy!

Vanilla Avocado Almond Smoothie

Ingredients

- 1/2 Avocado
- 1 tbsp almond butter
- 1/2 cup half and half or cream
- 1/2 cup unsweetened vanilla almond milk
- dash of ceylon cinnamon
- splash of vanilla extract or sugar free vanilla syrup
- 3/4 cup of ice
- no carb liquid sweetener to taste- STEVIA! :)

DIRECTIONS

Mix all together and enjoy!

Thanks again for checking out my book. I hope you enjoy these recipes and more importantly I hope these recipes will help you on your Ketogenic Journey and Lifestyle!